The Pocket Guide to Facial Enhancement Acupuncture

Paul Adkins

Acknowledgements

Thanks to my wife Karen for all of her support and help with this book, and also my thanks to Joan for being such a good friend and reliable demonstration patient.

Table of Contents

1
Introduction to Facial Enhancement Acupuncture

Before we begin I had better tell you a little bit about myself and where I am coming from. I studied 5 Element Acupuncture at the CTA Leamington College of 5 Element Acupuncture and gained an honors degree as well as the license to practice.

Since then I have been in practice treating my patients with 5 Element Acupuncture and developing Facial Enhancement Acupuncture.

The Facial element to my practice has developed rapidly over the last couple of years and I have now completed many hundreds of treatments. My other great pleasure in my working life is conducting workshops for other practitioners who are interested in the work I am doing.

These workshops started as very intimate affairs of 3 or 4 practitioners but have now grown to larger gatherings of a dozen or more students. We go through the techniques that I use on my own patients and discuss the use of Facial Enhancement Acupuncture in their own practices and clinics.

I have now conducted workshops in the UK and also abroad and have had practitioners from as far a field as the Middle East attend workshops at my clinic in Cornwall.

Most of my time these days is spent conducting these workshops although I do have regular patients that I see in my clinic. I am continually looking at ways to develop Facial

Enhancement Acupuncture and am always researching new techniques that I can use in my treatment protocol. At the moment I am investigating the use of Electro-Acupuncture in my practice. This is a field that is very new to me but something that I am very excited about and the results that I have been achieving are looking very promising - no doubt that will be something to cover in a subsequent edition of this Guide.

This book has been prompted by many friends and colleagues telling me that I should sit down and write this so having always done as I am told I have decided to do just that. What I am trying to convey to the reader is a background behind the techniques and protocols that have proven successful for me. One of the main points that I want to reiterate is that this type of Acupuncture should only be administered by qualified Acupuncturists and should never be undertaken by anyone who has not had the relevant Acupuncture training. While the points and techniques are well described in these pages this is no substitute for the practical experience of a hands on workshop so it would be nice to see as many of you as possible on one of my workshops in the future.

Another issue that I would like to clarify before we commence is that I do not profess to be the expert on everything Facial, I will try and explain to the best of my ability the methods and techniques that I know work for me. I do know the techniques that I have used on so many of my patients really do work and I have had some fantastic feedback from the patients that have received treatments. I cannot always give you the scientific data to back up my results, perhaps that is something someone else may like to research in the future.

With this style of Acupuncture it is very similar to other complimentary therapies in the way that it is very hard to put into words and quantify its results. What I can give you is an exciting treatment plan that will gain you many new patients who will be interested in not only your Facial Enhancement Acupuncture but also Acupuncture of all kinds whatever discipline you have trained in. When I started to think about names for the type of Acupuncture that I practice Enhancement is really what came to mind first. We are taking the

patient's appearance and enhancing the beauty that everyone has in their expressions, mannerisms and of course their
smile.

I am not one of those people who think we should eradicate
all signs of age from our patient's face; instead we should
celebrate the fact that someone has reached a certain age
and maturity in their life.

That's all very well and good I can hear you saying, but we
want to look younger and more attractive as well as being
older and wiser, fair enough, let's see how we can go about
helping our patients to do just that grow older looking and
feeling more vibrant than they have ever felt before.

Like many other Acupuncturists, I focus on a patient's well
being and inner harmony. To start talking about working on
the face and how a person looks probably goes against the
grain of how we look at Acupuncture. You have probably
been taught, as I have, that we are working with the mind,
body and spirit and not the physical looks of our patient.
However, my answer is that in the society we live in today,
people will always be looking for a way to look and feel better
about themselves.

As practitioners we know how terrific Acupuncture is, so why
not use it to help a patient with all aspects of their well being
both physical and emotional. Far better a patient comes to a
highly qualified professional such as yourself rather than try a
magic potion or visit some therapist who has only been qualified in their profession through a couple of weekend courses.

We all know that Acupuncture is natural and works with the
patients own Qi, so let's help a patient feel better about the
way they look as well, by using this wonderful system of
treatment. Many practitioners have asked me if I get as much
pleasure and enjoyment practicing Facial Enhancement
Acupuncture as using the skills I have learnt using my 5
Element practice. I usually answer that I do not make any
distinction between the two, it is all Acupuncture to me and it
helps patients feel better about themselves so in my mind
that's what it's all about.

THE POCKET GUIDE TO FACIAL ENHANCEMENT ACUPUNCTURE

What is very interesting to note is that out of all the patients that come to see me for Facial Enhancement Acupuncture probably 80% remain patients for 5 Element treatment after their course of Facial Enhancement Acupuncture have ended. That either says a lot for my skills and personality, or I think it is more likely to say how turned on to Acupuncture they have become, once they experience it for the first time whether it is Facial or Traditional Acupuncture.

So that's enough about me, now let's turn our attention to Facial Enhancement Acupuncture and what results your patients can expect from a course of treatments. The main benefit that you will find almost instantly is that your patient's general skin condition and skin tone will improve. If you are inserting thirty plus needles into the face you are bound to be affecting the circulation and the Qi energy throughout the skin. I have noticed a dramatic improvement in skin tone which becomes more even across the whole face and pores around the T zone of the nose and forehead do begin to shrink and close up. As we age the skin loses its elasticity and its ability to bounce back into shape and areas of the face start to sag, Facial Enhancement Acupuncture helps to tighten the underlying Facial muscles and hence reduce this sagging which can be more noticeable around the jowls of the patient.

When we look at a patient who has lots of lines around their eyes I personally do not see a great problem, these are evidence of character and a life lived to the full. However, they are not for everyone so at least with this type of Acupuncture we can effectively begin to reduce the appearance of these lines and also the bags and dark patches that appear under the eyes. One of my favourite areas of the face that I like to work on is the nasal labial fold; this is the crease that runs from the corner of the mouth to the side of the nose. Using the intradermal needling technique described later in these pages we can alter the appearance of this fold after only a few treatments.

Please bear in mind that a lot of what I am describing to you, you will already know as an experienced Acupuncturist. What I am trying to achieve by Facial Enhancement Acupuncture is a structure to the treatment and to compile the points and techniques into one easy treatment plan.

P.S. If like me you are a magpie for collecting Acupuncture books you will probably have rows of hard back journals and glossy publications taking up shelf space.

There are even some blank pages at the back of the book to make notes of new points you decide to use or any special tips that you want to remind yourself of - so please use it I expect to see it dog eared and creased after a few months of use.

This pocket guide was designed exactly as that, a pocket guide for regular reference.

The Muscles of the Face

Facial Enhancement Acupuncture works with the patient in many different ways. There is the spiritual side of an Acupuncture treatment and there are also the physical benefits to the skin through stimulation of Qi, which generates new skin growth and improves the circulation to the face.

With Facial Enhancement Acupuncture we are working with the various muscles in the face. Needles are used to stimulate the muscle and tighten them very similar to doing a sit up in the gym, the difference being we are training the muscles of the face, so we lose that sagginess that seems to plague us all as we age - actually having tried this on myself it is a lot easier than trying to get a six pack. It is useful to list the muscles of the face and neck; this will give you a chance to visualise the muscles when you needle.

Muscles of the Face:

Sternocleidomastoid - a pair of muscles running down either side of the neck. Helps to lift the head and also rotates the head sideways

The Eye Muscles:

Corrugator supercilii - this muscle pulls the eyebrows together in a frown. Frontalis raises the eyebrows

Orbicularis oculi - narrows the eyes to a squint

Procerus - pulls the eyebrows down and together

The Nose Muscles:
Depressor septi - depresses the nostrils
Levator labii superioris - flares the nostrils

The Mouth Muscles:
Buccinator - helps form the cheeks to blow a kiss
Depressor anguli oris - makes the lips grimace
Depressor labii inferioris - makes the lips pout
Levator labii superioris - opens the lips
Mentalis - wrinkles the chin
Orbicularis oris - helps the lips form a whistle sound
Platysma draws the corner of the mouth down
Risorius - helps the mouth form a grin
Zygmaticus major and Zygomaticus minor lifts the mouth to smile

Muscles of the Jaw:
Masseter - clenches the teeth together
Temporalis - raises the lower jaw when chewing

What results can I expect?
This is obviously one of the first questions that a prospective patient will ask. They have been intrigued by the idea of a Facial treatment that does not involve invasive surgery and they are fascinated by a natural approach to the way we look within the beauty industry.

I always stress to my students to give a patient a realistic expectation. It is of no benefit to you or them to make false claims and promises which will only lead to disappointment in the long run.

However, having said, that it still amazes me the astonishing results that have been achieved by using the points I describe for Facial treatments. The first thing a patient will notice after their first treatment is the improvement to the tone and texture of their skin, the Qi energy that is generated in the face during a treatment will show itself very early on and after a few days the patient should have a radiant glow that is very evident to people around them.

INTRODUCTION TO FACIAL ENHANCEMENT ACUPUNCTURE

Many patients report back to me after treatment and say that their friends have noticed they are looking well but cannot put their finger on what is different about them. Working with the facial muscles and the contours of the face to achieve a structural change can take a little longer but even after only two or three treatments the patient should notice a dramatic reduction in fine lines and also any puffiness that may be apparent on the face. The pores will tighten and a more even colour and tone should be evident across the face.

For longer term changes to the patient's appearance it will be necessary to conduct treatment on a regular basis, when and at what intervals can obviously vary from patient to patient depending on their individual circumstances. However, you will notice very dramatic results as the muscles in the face tighten and the lines and wrinkles start to fade.

In my own practice I have had patients that come for a one off treatment before a special occasion and I have some patients who I treat every couple of weeks and will probably do so for as long as they keep coming. Both you and your patients will be amazed at the results that can be achieved by selective use of Acupuncture points on the face. As practicing Acupuncturists this shouldn't come as any surprise at all as we have known for a long time the awesome power of Acupuncture.

What should I charge?
During this introduction you may have noticed that I have not mentioned charges that I make to my patients/clients. I use both patient and client as I am still not sure how to address them, I think I will stick to patients as this is a term I am familiar with and fits in with the whole ethos of what I am doing. There are many factors to consider when deciding what to charge. The location of your clinic and your own personal overheads will dictate how much you decide to charge your patients and this may vary from practitioner to practitioner.

I make no mention as to the amount of treatments that I would recommend for a patient. It is obvious that someone who has only a couple of treatments will not show the same results as a patient who embarks on a course of six or more. I consider each patient individually and gauge my treatment plan to suit there own specific needs. One thing I will stress make sure your prices reflect the hard work that a treatment involves and don't forget that you are using lots of high quality needles when conducting your treatments.

Never let the subject of fees or cost become an embarrassment to you. As a qualified Acupuncturist you have trained for many years to perfect your techniques and understanding of Chinese medicine. You are now offering your patients a new level of treatment that takes you into a totally different market place. Thousands of dollars and pounds are spent each day on beauty and cosmetic procedures throughout the world and patients think nothing of spending large amounts on individual procedures. As a Facial Enhancement Acupuncturist you are now able to offer a natural and safe alternative and you should be rewarded for doing that.

I have known many very successful Acupuncturists who make a very good living out of their knowledge and expertise. I have also known many who struggle and find they need to work at other jobs in order to make ends meet. If you decide to offer Facial Enhancement Acupuncture from your clinic you will find a whole new customer base opens up to you which will enable you to pay those bills and earn the type of living that you deserve.

Who can have Facial Enhancement Acupuncture?
Almost anyone can benefit from Facial Enhancement Acupuncture, However, as with any Acupuncture treatment there are a few conditions, that when confronted with, I would examine if I wanted to proceed with a course of treatment. I would definitely look very closely at carrying out a treatment with a patient who experiences high blood pressure or has had problems with their blood clotting in the past.

If a patient has been diagnosed with cancer or coronary disease then my usual precautions would be taken as with any normal Acupuncture procedure. The emphasis should be on common sense when dealing with your patient. If there are underlying issues that make the patient unhappy with their appearance then whatever you do as a practitioner will not make them happy. It might be in everyone's interest to address these issues before treatment commences.

At this point this is where your extensive Acupuncture knowledge comes into play. Imagine a patient going to a consultant for another type of cosmetic procedure. If there were underlying problems that the patient was suffering with, that consultant may not have the expertise or experience to deal with them.

As an Acupuncturist you can support and nurture the patient in so many ways. After having had Traditional Acupuncture with you for any underlying issues, the patient may decide that they do not wish to carry on with Facial Enhancement Acupuncture. This is fine, you still have a new patient and better still you have a more balanced patient. As with any Acupuncture treatment I am always conscious to look out for any indications that may need me to refer the patient onto a medical practitioner and this applies the same with my Facial procedure. If at anytime I am aware of the symptoms or conditions of an illness that cause me any concern then I will always refer the patient on to a medical consultant.

Needles and equipment required

If you are anything like me you are probably an equipment junkie. I love having the latest tools of the trade and a drawer full of gadgets. If this is the case then Facial Enhancement Acupuncture is for you. When you start to offer this type of Acupuncture from your clinic you will soon notice that you start to accumulate pieces of equipment that you never thought you would use during an Acupuncture treatment. Take a look at the list of essential items and you will understand what I mean.

As an Acupuncturist we each have our own preference as to the type of needle that we like to use. My recommendations here are purely taken from my own experiences of carrying out hundreds of Facial Enhancement Acupuncture treatments. I have always preferred to use metal handled needles for Acupuncture on body points but have found that plastic handle needles are far better for Facial work as the lightness of their construction means they do not fall over onto the face. The brand of needle that I use has colour coded handles for the different gauges of shaft, this is ideal as you can plan different parts of your treatment according to the color needle you are using.

The quality of needle used is of the utmost importance. During a Facial treatment you can use up to 30 needles on the face and it is essential that the finest gauge needles you are able to work with are used. As well as the standard Acupuncture needles that are used in a Facial treatment we also use Japanese intradermal needles. Some Acupuncturists are not that familiar with these needles but I have found them to be one of the most useful products that I have ever discovered. I have been so impressed with these needles that I now use them in my Acupuncture practice for treating back and shoulder problems.

Listed overleaf, are some of the items of equipment that are needed to carry out a Facial Enhancement Acupuncture treatment, obviously you will have your own preferences and this list should be treated only as a guide until you find out what suits you best.

At the end of the book you will find a section where I have listed some useful contact details; this list includes suppliers where you can purchase all of the needles that I recommend to use, both of the suppliers that I use regularly are very helpful and if you have any questions they are always ready to help.

Essential items of equipment for a Facial Enhancement Acupuncture treatment

1" Finest Quality 14 gauge needles
½" Finest Quality 14 gauge needles
3mm Intradermal needles
6mm Intradermal needles
1" Metal handle needles
Good quality square nosed tweezers
Small magnet
Cotton wool buds
Arnica cream or capsules

INTRODUCTION TO FACIAL ENHANCEMENT ACUPUNCTURE

Facial massage oil or cream (this is covered in a later section of the book)
Small hand mirror
Make up remover or wipes
Cotton wool
Medi-wipes
Hand cleansing gel

As a practicing acupuncturist you will already be familiar with some of the items that I have listed on the previous page. However, I am sure you are already perplexed as to the use of a magnet and also massage oil, at this stage don't let this worry you too much, we will go into greater depth with regard to these items as we progress through the different stages of treatment.

Treatment Room and Initial Consultation
This subject is as vast as you like to make it and people will question why I need to mention it at all. The reason for my inclusion of a section on the treatment room is that I have seen many therapists' treatment rooms and equipment and they vary enormously according to the character and practice of the Acupuncturist. I was very much brought up under the 5 Element school of teaching so I would never have used fragrances in my room otherwise these would mask the diagnostics of odour, and to play music in the treatment room would definitely not be in order. Most practice rooms that I have seen are quite basic and not particularly cheery places to work in.
Sometimes this is down to the fact that many treatment rooms are in private practices and are shared by a few practitioners in the building. This does make it difficult to personalise the room but I have still seen some terrific treatment rooms that are used by a few practitioners.
The first thing I would say to any practitioner embarking on Facial Enhancement Acupuncture is to schedule your Facial treatments on a different day to your general Acupuncture. As you will see as we progress the approach to Facial En-

hancement Acupuncture is totally different to other Acupuncture and I feel is a different mind set altogether.

I find it very welcoming for my patients if I am playing music in my clinic very similar to a visit to a therapist for a massage or pampering session. I also like to have some type of relaxing incense burning in the room, these are things that I would not normally do when carrying out a general Acupuncture treatment, but are quite acceptable for the type of Facial treatment that we are carrying out.

When a patient enquires about Facial Enhancement Acupuncture for the first time I generally like to meet them for an initial consultation where we can discuss their expectations of treatment and also their commitment to a treatment programme. This initial meeting is crucial to the ongoing patient practitioner relationship, similar to a traditional treatment plan in the more mainstream Acupuncture treatments.

What I have found to be a lot more important in this type of relationship are the reasons behind the patient wanting to have treatment. In this day and age when expectations of how we should look are forced upon us from every direction we need to make sure that the patient is embarking on a treatment plan for all the right reasons and not just media pressure and hype.

It is important as with any traditional Acupuncture consultation not to feel pressurised to take a patient on if you do not feel they are suitable or ready for treatment, or their expectations of treatment are far greater than can be achieved by the protocol you are offering. Don't be afraid to turn a patient away if you are not comfortable with treating them.

We can achieve some staggering results using Facial Enhancement Acupuncture but there is obviously a limit to anything that we do. During this initial consultation it may also become obvious that the patient needs some other form of treatment before Facial Enhancement Acupuncture treatment can commence.

It may be necessary to enter into some agreement with the patient that they commit to a series of Traditional Acupuncture treatments before you will undertake the Facial Enhancement Acupuncture.

This is where the hand mirror we talked about earlier comes into use. Have the patient look into the mirror and have them point out what they would like to achieve from treatment. It is very important that at this stage the practitioner makes a note somewhere of these requests so they can refer back to them during the course of treatment and point out the results to the patient. What you will find with patients is that they are never totally happy with the results they will always end up convincing themselves that they look the same or nothing has changed. When this happens you need to be able to get out the notes you made at the initial meeting and remind them of how things were then and point out the progression since that first meeting.

Some students have asked me about using before and after photographs of my patients, this is not something that I do myself but I have no real problem with it either, I will leave it up to you. You need to make sure the conditions are right for both the before and after photography for example, the lighting, seating colouring of the backdrop otherwise trying to make a comparison could be difficult.

During the consultation the subject of price will arise, if this hasn't been discussed beforehand. As stated earlier, pricing is down to the individual practitioner. However I would urge that you ensure to charge enough taking into account your expertise, time and the equipment you are using. It is advisable to have the patient commit to a series of treatments. Although they will benefit from a one off procedure, the effects of this treatment are cumulative and the results will really start to show after 3-4 treatments. By showing commitment to a series of treatments shows how keen the patient is.

I have found by offering a discount to patients who pay for say a course of 12 treatments in advance a very good way of filling the diary and also generating some cash flow. Although I would not object to treating a patient on a one off basis, I would generally insist that they commence a course of at least twelve treatments, this way I know that I am going to be able to give them the results that they are looking for and after the course of treatment I would then generally recommend that a patient has a top up procedure every month or so.

At this stage it is also worth pointing out to the patient that some bruising can occur during and after a treatment and that this is normal and should not be a concern. The bruising should settle down after a couple of days and if a bruise does occur when you are carrying out a treatment the first thing to do is not to panic. Have some arnica cream ready to apply to the area it might be worth applying some light pressure to the bruise especially if it is a small lump, this can be done by using a cotton bud. If done soon enough this should stop a bruise developing.

The answer really is to warn your patient in advance of the possibility, that way they will not get a shock if a bruise occurs. If a patient has a special occasion coming up I would probably not treat them within a couple of days of that date - it would be awful to give a patient a black eye on the day before their wedding. To avoid these types of problems I always advise my students to be positive and confident with their needle technique, if you are confident and practiced in what you do you will find that bruising is not really an issue.

2
The Facial Enhancement Acupuncture 10 Steps Treatment

These are some of the Acupuncture points we use during a treatment (no particular order). This list is by no means the only points that are used; it is merely a guide as to the points that come up more regularly during a treatment. There may be points that you discover yourself as you conduct your treatments which you can add to the list.

Liver 3
Stomach 36
Spleen 9
Gall Bladder 41
Stomach 44
Large Intestine 4
Triple Heater 8
Pericardium 4
Shen Men
Stomach 13
Gall Bladder 21
Triple Heater 15
Stomach 9
Governor Vessel 20
Bladder 6
Gall Bladder 14

Bladder 2
Triple Heater 23
YuYao
Stomach 5
Stomach 4
Stomach 3
Small Intestine 18
Large intestine 19
Ren 23
Ren 24
Small Intestine 17
Triple Heater 17

The 10 Steps Treatment

Step: 1   AE or detox procedure. Needle the feet and legs
Step: 2   Needle the hand points
Step: 3   Auricular points
Step: 4   Neck area stage, depending on requirements of the patient
Step: 5   Working on the head and face
Step: 6   Needle the chin and cheek areas
Step: 7   Check the control needles in the patients hand and arm
Step: 8   Front of face
Step: 9   Intradermal needling
Step: 10 Facial massage and assess the results ready for the next treatment

The full Facial Enhancement Acupuncture treatment
Step 1:

How we start a treatment is very much down to the preferences of the practitioner. It is important that before we embark on a series of treatments we perform some sort of detox or clearing treatment on the patient.

Because of my 5 Element background and training the obvious choice for me would be to perform an aggressive energy drain on the patient, this is a particular treatment protocol found in 5 Element practice. However depending on your Acupuncture background this could be an Auricular detox or other clearing treatment that you may specialise in. Again depending on your school of Acupuncture I would take the patient's pulses and also investigate their general health condition before starting the treatments. When the patient has settled on the couch and is relaxed, I would begin the treatment.

I should also mention that when you carry out a Facial Enhancement Acupuncture treatment you are lent over the patient for a great deal of the time I would definitely invest in a comfortable stool of the appropriate height that you can work from behind the patient's head and lean over their face, this will prevent you from straining your back. It is very useful to have a good source of light at the head end of your couch that way the fine needle work that is required during a treatment will not put a strain on your eyes. When needling the patient they should be horizontal on the couch with some light head support giving you free access to the patient's face and neck.

I always start to needle the points on the patient's feet and legs first. These points are designed to give a good grounding for the treatment and should always be needled.

The temptation to skip this step of the treatment should never be given in to. The points on the feet are needled bi-laterally and needled with an evens technique (neither tonified or sedated) these needles are retained throughout the treatment and are the last needles to be removed.

LV3 Tai Chong (Supreme Rushing) this is a lovely Earth point which used in conjunction with LI4 is part of the four gates treatment, one of the uses of this treatment is to Expel wind from the face.

ST36 Zu San Li (Leg Three Miles) A very important point, a lovely enriching point for Mind, Body and Spirit.

SP9 Yin Ling Quan (Yin Mound Spring) Water He-Sea point.

GB41 Zu Lin Qi (Foot above Tears) Wood Point, this is an important point due to its connection with the eyes.

ST44 Nei Ting (Inner Courtyard) A great point again used in conjunction with LI4 to expel wind from the face, also has uses as an analgesia point for tooth extractions.

The points that I have described to be used on the patient's feet and legs are by no means written in stone, they are the points that from experience I have found benefit the patient most, also a couple of the points are used in the four gates treatment protocol.

As Acupuncturists we all have favourite points that from experience, we like to use also as we know points vary from patient to patient. There is no reason that you should not include points of your own choice in this part of the treatment.

Step: 2

After needling the points on the feet and legs we then move to points on the patient's hands and forearm. These three points are probably some of the most powerful points that I use. Used primarily as pain relief points in this treatment, although pain may be too strong a term here and it is more accurate to say discomfort, these points are therefore stimulated during the treatment procedure.

As Acupuncturists you should be familiar with the anesthetic qualities of these points and that their combination is frequently used in China for anesthetic during some quite major surgical procedures. The Chinese journal of Acupuncture refers to the practice of needling through the arm to needle both TH8 and PC4 in one movement. I really think we ought to give that technique a miss so let's just use the two needles for the time being. Again do not be tempted to skip this step of the treatment the power of these points cannot be underestimated and will help with your patient's well being during the Facial Enhancement Acupuncture treatment.

We will discuss later in this book the fact that I do not attempt to achieve the sensation of Da-Qi on any Acupuncture point that we use on the face or neck. However, it is important that the sensation of Da-Qi is achieved and maintained when needling the points on the hand and forearm, again needle these points bi-laterally.

LI4 He Gu (Joining of the Valleys) this is probably my favourite Acupuncture point; I find I use it in so many of my treatments.

TH8 San Yang Luo (Three Yang Junction) Used in Conjunction with PC4 as an anesthetic point.

PC4 Xi Men, Hsiman (Gate of Qi Reserve) Used as an analgesic point with TH8.

THE FACIAL ENHANCEMENT ACUPUNCTURE 10 STEPS TREATMENT

We have already mentioned the subject of Acupuncture and Anesthesia, during the Facial Enhancement Acupuncture treatment I always use the points LI4 (Joining of the valleys) TH8 (Sanyanglo) and PC4 (Hsimen). The thought behind the use of these points is to assist the patient with any discomfort that they may feel from the treatment, this is particularly important if the patient is new to Acupuncture and not really sure what to expect.

At this point if you want to you can skip this section and move on to the next step of the treatment plan, alternatively if you are like me and find anything Acupuncture related interesting you may like to read on and look into Acupuncture and pain relief in greater depth.

The focus of this chapter is to look at the role of Acupuncture Anesthesia in Chinese Medicine, and to start to explore the reasons why this type of practice has not developed in the Western hemisphere. This investigation has looked at the classical texts, literature from medical institutions, the theory of Five Element Acupuncture and also Western publications. There was a great deal written on the subject of Acupuncture Anesthesia during the early 1970s. However, after this initial enthusiasm for the subject the interest in the West subsided and very little was reported in Western literature or medical journals.

The interest in the practice of this particular form of medicine developed and continued to be used extensively in China and countries such as Japan and Korea, to the point where it is still in use today in the majority of Chinese hospitals.

I have always been fascinated by the use of Acupuncture as an instrument in the relief of pain. This subject stirs the imagination and statements, such as the one by Duke, and adds fuel to the intrigue of the subject.

"With a number of Canadian diplomats watching, a doctor performed delicate open-heart surgery. As he held a human heart in his hand, the wide awake woman patient sipped orange juice" (Duke 1972 p5.)

What has interested me most about this form of Acupuncture is that pain is present in Eastern Medicine as well as Western Medicine, so why has this proven method of pain relief not developed in our Western society?

19

Perhaps what is thought by many as an Eastern tradition is okay for the Chinese but would not be acceptable to the West as described by Lewith.

"One of the main criticisms of Acupuncture Anesthesia is that 'it's alright for the Chinese, but won't work on Europeans'. Acupuncture Anesthesia has been used in a variety of European Centers and the success and failure rate is much the same as in China. Acupuncture Anesthesia is a useful method of pain relief and could well be applicable to minor procedures, or post-operative pain relief, within the context of a Western medical system."
(Lewith 2003.)

An argument that can be raised, to justify the lack of development of Acupuncture Anesthesia development in Western medicine, is that this type of medical procedure is relatively new to our society and has not had the benefit of thousands of years of use, as is the case in China. This, however, would be a misconception as Acupuncture has, of course, been in existence for thousands of years, but as described by Chen (1973) in "Acupuncture Anesthesia in the peoples republic of China, 1973". It was not until 1958 that the technique of Acupuncture Anesthesia was created in modern China. The idea that this form of Anesthesia was only adopted in the middle of the 20th century is, of course, misleading and perhaps should be phrased differently adding in its present form.

There are references to the use of Acupuncture as an analgesic which go back many hundreds of years, for example, in the translation "The Yellow Emperors Classic of internal Medicine" Veith (1972) the author describes the medical records of an eminent Chinese surgeon, who in the second century BC were said to have exchanged the hearts of two patients using Acupuncture as part of the anesthetic.

Another well known figure from Chinese history was the so called "Father of surgery". This was *Hua Tuo* (110-207AD), and it is well described in the publication "In the footsteps of the Yellow emperor" Eckman (1996) how *Hua Tuo* was the physician to emperor *Cao Cao* and although he did demonstrate mastery of Acupuncture with the insertion of very few needles he was also the inventor of a method of Anesthesia using Chinese herbs which he incorporated into his Acupuncture treatments. Unfortunately for *Hua Tao* the emperor was not impressed when he was diagnosed as having a brain tumor and proceeded to have the physician decapitated at the age of 97.

It has been said that Acupuncture Anesthesia *(Zhenci masui)* or Acuanalgesia as the procedure is also sometimes known, bears no relationship to Acupuncture other than the fact that both techniques employ the use of needles, this may be a wildly exaggerated view but none the less is a view that has been expressed by some people.

These thoughts are expressed in "Chinese Medicine its history" Porkert and Ullman (1982) the description of needle technique in general Acupuncture and that of the technique in Acupuncture Anesthesia does vary greatly. There is a far greater stimulation of the needle for Anesthesia purposes and this can involve a twirling motion or a thrusting action of the needle, this is in stark contrast to the more sensitive stimulation of the point during a general Acupuncture treatment. The selection of points also used in Anesthesia treatment bears less and less resemblance to the points used throughout the history of Chinese Acupuncture.

"Chinese Medicine its history" Porkert and Ullman (1982) illustrate this decline in the resemblance of Acupuncture Anesthesia to the origins of Traditional Acupuncture and its theory and practice.

"So that eventually there may appear to be absolutely no connection whatever with classical theory or practice."
(Porkert and Ullman 1982 p 229.)

As Acupuncture Anesthesia has developed throughout the centuries, more recently the idea of stimulation to the needle other than that which would normally occur during a standard Acupuncture treatment has also developed. This stimulation can now be induced by electrical current which has the same affect on the patient as the original twirling and thrusting of the needle as described earlier.

This more aggressive needle technique, which developed and later became an integral part of the TCM style of practice, is described in "Understanding Acupuncture" Birch (1999) this was the technique that Western visitors to China were shown and which was taken back and incorporated into Western Medicine.

This aggressive needle stimulation and action was later carried out by the use of electrical stimulation. This area of Acupuncture has become a specialist field in its own right.

The practice of electro Acupuncture is well described in "Mechanisms of electro-Acupuncture analgesia as related to endorphins and monoamines; an intricate system is proposed"Shing Sou Cheng (1980) he goes into great detail of the equipment and procedures that are employed in this type of treatment. It is the author's intention to explore electro Acupuncture later in this study.

The early procedures that were conducted in the 1950's were for conditions such as toothache and tonsillectomy, and these were conducted by medical workers from the *Sian, Shanghai* and *Hopei* provinces. These minor procedures then developed into more significant surgical operations as the knowledge of Anesthesia and its affects were developed This development is well documented in the work " Acupuncture Anesthesia in the peoples republic of China, 1973"
Chen (1973).

The first actual successful medical trial in the early 1950s was as anesthetic in a tonsillectomy operation. The success of this procedure made way for rapid development of the technique, whereby originally Acupuncture points on the body and limbs were used but this quickly developed into the use of points on the ear, face and the nose. Early procedure relied on a number of practitioners each stimulating points on the patient; this could require the use of up to

Eighty different points, eventually as knowledge and experience was developed this number of points was dramatically reduced to only a few needles.

As described in great detail in "Acupuncture Anesthesia in the peoples republic of China, 1973" Chen (1973) it is believed that an analgesic effect can be achieved by the use of two points when conducting a Tonsillectomy procedure, the author has listed these points using their Five Element Acupuncture names as we know them, the points used in this operation are *"LI4*

Joining of the Valleys and TH6 Branch Ditch" (College of traditional Acupuncture 2000). These points would be needled bilaterally.

These surgical developments were of a profound medical influence which also had political backing and were instigated by *Mao Tse Tung* the leader of the Chinese people at the time. This development of Acupuncture Anesthesia was his idea of East meeting West in surgical procedures and is described in "Acupuncture in Anesthesia" Streitberger (2003). I was intrigued by the selection of LI4 and TH6 as the chosen points that would aid in the analgesic affect, required to perform the tonsillectomy procedure, but what was the significance in the choice of these point to the many other points that could have been chosen? A very clear and concise description of points and their indications can be found in "A Manual of Acupuncture" Deadman and Al-Khafaji (2001). The Large Intestine channel extends from the tip of the index finger along the arm and ends at the side of the nose, along this journey the channel extends through the neck, this extension through the neck may be of particular interest in the case of tonsillectomy as the Large Intestine channel has always been found to have analgesic affects at all of the points along the meridian, they are particularly good at regulating *Qi* and Blood and treating obstructions and pain of all kinds.

The significance of the use of the Triple Heater *(San Jiao)* channel is again interesting in the context of the tonsillectomy procedure, this channel starts at the tip of the ring finger again travels across the neck and finishes alongside the outer canthus of the eye. The Triple Heater official is responsible for the regulation of heat and temperature throughout the body. This is very significant as in the case of tonsillitis there is a great deal of inflammatory heat present. In the publication "A Manual of Acupuncture" Deadman and Al-Khafaji (2001) describe the Triple Heater channel as the channel that belongs to fire and is responsible for fever in the body, also how use of the points on this channel can clear heat from the neck, throat and tongue.

The point that is used with the most success on the *San Jiao* channel for treatment of tonsillitis is Triple Heater 6 *(Branch Ditch)*, this point is located on the forearm between the radius and the ulna bones, it has many actions associated to it but ones of particular interest with regard to this condition are its benefits in clearing heat and also it aids the voice.

Another relatively simple procedure but one that affects most people is tooth extraction, the Acupuncture Anesthesia protocols for this procedure are well documented in "Acupuncture Anesthesia in the peoples republic of China, 1973" Chen (1973). What is interesting is the accuracy of the points relating to which teeth are to be extracted, also the idea that finger pressure on the appropriate point will provide enough analgesic affect to carry on with the extraction.

Chen (1973) " Acupuncture Anesthesia in the peoples republic of China, 1973" describes his astonishment to be present and witness tooth extractions that were carried out painlessly in a few minutes using only acupressure techniques.

While I find such examples of Acupuncture treatments to be very impressive, something that really did grab my attention was the description of a patient who was about to undergo abdominal surgery with Acupuncture as the only Anesthesia. This was very well documented and illustrated in "Acupuncture" Duke (1972) how is it feasible that a patient can remain awake and alert while having a major surgical procedure conducted on them.

One of these procedures described in "Acupuncture" Duke (1972) really conjured the imagination of the author, it describes a doctor holding the heart of a patient in his hand while she sips orange juice and apparently feels no discomfort from the operation due to the Acupuncture Anesthesia that is being administered to her.

This very dangerous operation had been conducted with the patient completely aware of what was going on. This had the obvious benefits to the patient that there were not the risks that can be associated with conventional anesthetic also the advantages to the surgeon were clear in the way that he could communicate with the patient during the procedure and thus gauge her condition and response to the operation, and of course one of the most significant advantages was the quick recovery time from a very serious procedure. With all of these obvious advantages that we have discussed, this again prompts to ask the question as to why this type of procedure has not developed within Western Medicine; this is something I must continue to investigate. While it is easy to be amazed by these surgical procedures that show a patient wide awake and lucid while having lung surgery, it must always be understood that there are disadvantages to this type of procedure.

Now is probably a good time for me to look at some of the potential problems that can arise. In his publication "Acupuncture Anesthesia in the peoples republic of China, 1973" Chen (1973) goes into some detail about the potential difficulties that can arise when conducting a surgical procedure using Acupuncture as the anesthetic.

There are three main disadvantages as outlined in "Acupuncture Anesthesia in the people's republic of China, 1973" Chen (1973). These are described as incomplete analgesia, inadequate muscular relaxation and incomplete control of internal visceral response. Acupuncture Anesthesia must not be looked upon as a total replacement for normal surgical procedures but rather as a compliment to the normal medical preparation for a surgical operation, this is very well described in "Medical Acupuncture applications in Surgical Anesthesia" Mock (2000) which discusses the role of pre-operative preparation for surgery with Acupuncture.

The benefits of this type of Anesthesia become particularly relevant when we are dealing with older patients to whom there would be greater risks using conventional anesthetic procedures.

Dr Wen, "Orthopedic surgery on the elbow", describes a procedure that involves the placing of nails and other hardware into the Olecranon of a female patient who is well into her sixties. This operation would be termed high risk using general anesthetic but using Acupuncture the surgeon is able to bring on an analgesic affect by the stimulation of only two points Heart 1 and Large Intestine 17, these two points are on either side of the Brachial nerve and were enough to produce enough analgesic affect for the operation to take place.

If we go from one end of the age spectrum back to the other we can look at surgery in children while using Acupuncture as the anesthetic. The benefits of this type of procedure on children is that, in many cases, it would be beneficial to have feedback from the patient during or directly after the procedure, in the case of Acupuncture Anesthesia this remains possible as the patient is conscious throughout.

"Acupuncture Augmentation of local Anesthesia with intravenous sedation for a child undergoing awake craniotomy", Schwartz (1998) shows dramatically how the benefits of Acupuncture Anesthesia and the fact that the patient remains conscious influences the success of a procedure, the description of a procedure on a 10 year old female patient provides evidence of the benefits when it is clear that the procedure could not have been undertaken under normal general Anesthetic. The success of any procedure that is carried out on young children would rely greatly on the pre-surgery briefing and the atmosphere that is generated in the operating room by the surgeon and his staff. As the patient remains conscious throughout, what could be a traumatic operation there needs to be the support in place to help the patient understand what is happening to them? The support and counseling that is required by the patient may be a factor in the lack of interest that is shown in the West for this type of procedure.

The Theories as to why Acupuncture can produce the analgesic affects that it does have been discussed for quite sometime, one of the theories behind the analgesic mechanism is the so called "Gate Theory" this theory is very clearly described in "The Web that has no Weaver-understanding Chinese Medicine" Kaptchuck (1983) this theory suggests that the stimulation that is delivered by the needles jams the nerve bundles in the central nervous system this prevents pain signals that may arise from incisions or surgery being sent to the brain.

"The Web that has no Weaver-understanding Chinese Medicine" Kaptchuck (1983) provides a very interesting interpretation of the central nervous system, likening it to a telephone system in a major city.

"This can be envisioned by imagining a telephone system in a major city: if too many individual lines are in use it is very difficult for an outside caller to get into the trunk lines and make a connection".
(Kaptchuck 1983)

THE FACIAL ENHANCEMENT ACUPUNCTURE 10 STEPS TREATMENT

Another theory that has been talked about regarding Acupuncture Anesthesia is that the insertion of the needles actually stimulates the body's endorphins; these are opiates that are produced within the brain. Opiates such as these are very potent painkillers and could be responsible for dulling the pain during a surgical procedure.

These are all very possible theories as to the success of Acupuncture Anesthesia when we look at the position of Acupuncture points and the directions the meridians run in, the points that are used very often are on meridians or channels that cross or flow to the affected areas.

What really puts a question mark upon these theories is when we look at Acupuncture Anesthesia in the context of Auricular Acupuncture, this is a form of Acupuncture that only uses points that are positioned on the ear to provide treatment for illness, this type of Acupuncture has always been very successful in the controlling of pain and particularly useful because of the analgesic affects that it produces. According to the publication "Handbook to Chinese Auricular therapy" Chen and Yongqiang (1991) the history of Auricular Acupuncture can be traced back as much as 4000 years ago when early Chinese texts described how certain channel systems converged upon the auricle.

They describe the ear as being the shape of an inverted fetus and there are points that are linked to the body's organs and functions situated all over the parts of the ear, these points can be stimulated manually or through electro Acupuncture to achieve the sensations that are required.

Auricular analgesia as it has become to be known has proven very successful as an addition to Western medical procedures, it is very easy to administer, as all points required are in a small area on the ear, and there is very little specialist equipment that is needed to promote the anesthetic affects. The fact that the patient remains conscious throughout the surgical procedure is of great benefit both during the operation and also in the recovery stages after the surgical procedure.

The use of Auricular Acupuncture is a favorable form of Acupuncture Anesthesia because of the state of mental alertness that the patient maintains this awareness of the patient ensures good communication between patient and surgeon, as described in "Handbook to Chinese Auricular therapy" Chen and Yongqiang (1991). Before any operation can take place using Auricular analgesia it is very important to have assessed the patient's tolerance to pain, also the condition of their *Qi* energy in the pre – operative period. If the patient is not totally responsive to the treatment and their commitment to the procedure is not total then the success of the procedure is in doubt, equally the patient must have total confidence in the surgeon and the team around him. In all cases of Acupuncture Anesthesia including, Auricular Analgesia, it is advisable to have a back-up plan in place that may involve more conventional anesthetics, should the Acupuncture cease to have any affect.

Because Auricular analgesia is specifically working on Acupuncture points of the ear, the selection and the stimulation of these points and their accuracy is crucial to achieve the desired levels of analgesic affect. Once the appropriate points have been selected the manipulation of these points is what achieves the analgesic stimulus, this manipulation can be hand manipulation and is only on a rotational basis as the ear is too thin to practice any thrusting stimulation.

The other type of stimulation is electro Acupuncture which involves passing a current through the needle to maintain stimulation throughout the surgical procedure, this can prove very successful although it is necessary to find the Acupuncture point by hand and insert the needles manually initially. Another benefit and use of Acupuncture Anesthesia, which is probably not so dramatic as the major surgical procedures that we have looked at so far, would be the use of Acupuncture Anesthesia as a treatment for minor traumas and also for paramedic support in awkward environments or conflict situations.

One of the most evident benefits of Acupuncture Anesthesia over more conventional anesthetics has to be the limited equipment that is necessary to conduct the procedure. It has been shown how the use of up to 80 needles were used in the early surgical operations, however, the development of point selection has reduced this to only two or three needles and in some cases the use of only one needle provides the analgesic response required. The lack of technical equipment and relative ease of use would lead the author to believe that this type of procedure would be ideal for treating the victims of trauma from conflict and hostile situations

All types of Acupuncture Anesthesia require some stimulation of the Acupuncture point. This is achieved by twirling or thrusting of the needle, initially this manipulation of the needle was done manually but as technology improved electro stimulation of the needle was developed; this procedure involves passing a variable electrical current through the needle which can be adjusted to produce the required stimulation for the point being treated.

This electro stimulation of the needle enabled longer stimulation of the needles than perhaps would have been possible using a manual technique but it is still necessary to find and stimulate the point manually so as to feel the patients *Qi* before electro stimulation can take over.

"Mechanisms of Electro Acupuncture analgesia as related to endorphins and monoamines; an intricate system is proposed" Cheng (1980) discusses the process of Electro Acupuncture and its ability to release Endorphins and Monoamines, his experiments on mice are well documented and evidenced.

When the needle is stimulated using an electrical current there is a pulsating sensation which the patient feels, this will be identical to the stimulation that is achieved by the manual manipulation of the needle. "Acupuncture Anesthesia in the peoples republic of China, 1973" Chen (1973) emphasizes the point that when using electro Acupuncture every effort should be made to achieve the sensation of *Te-Chi*.

The benefits of electrical stimulation of the needle in the procedures is obvious, the Anesthetic procedure can be carried out by far fewer practitioners as stimulation can remain constant by the intervention of the electrical pulses, but I still questions the sensations that are missing when the Acupuncture practitioner administers the stimulation and feels the *Te-chi* using there own hands. Electrical stimulation appears far more acceptable to Western medical practitioners than the manual stimulation of needles by the Acupuncture practitioner. I believe this acceptance is the case because the Western medical profession are far more likely to accept a procedure that relies on tangible equipment than a practice that involves a practitioner communicating with a patients *Qi* through his own hands and a needle which leans towards the more spiritual and mystic beliefs.

The subject of Acupuncture and pain relief is something that I will continue to investigate and develop its use in my Facial treatments, what I do know is that during the hundreds of Facial treatments that I have carried out I cannot remember a single patient complaining of any discomfort, it would be nice to think this was down to my needle technique but probably more likely the use of the powerful Acupuncture points.

Step: 3

Many acupuncturists that I know and have worked with are not that familiar with the points of the ear, unless of course they are an Auricular specialist. The Acupuncture points of the ear are some of the most powerful points and many practitioners achieve fantastic results with their patients by only using these points, in fact there are many successful acupuncturist who run only Auricular clinics. I will always use the point Shen men left then right for every treatment that I perform. Also in conjunction with the point Shen men I will choose to use another Auricular point that would correspond with a particular area of the face that I am keen to work on, there are many fine publications specializing in Auricular Acupuncture and they all seem to feature very accurate diagrams showing the many points on the ear, it may be worth purchasing one of these large wall charts for the wall of your clinic, this will give you an instant reference when deciding which point you should choose. For example this could be points such as mandible, cheek, or eye, or alternatively an organ point that you feel may be relevant to this particular patient. like to use the ½" 14 gauge needles for all Auricular work, these needles are an ideal size and are very easy to use, for those of you not familiar with the points on the ear have a cotton bud ready fro when you remove the needles as the ears do tend to bleed very easily.

I have listed 10 Auricular points that I use a lot in the treatments that I perform. There are no real reasons for choosing these points other than they are ones that are familiar to me, it would be foolhardy of me to try and go into too much detail about Auricular Acupuncture at this stage as it is a subject that requires research of its own. The points that I am recommending will be fine for the Facial treatments that you will be performing, but should you decide to do some more research there are many interesting book available on the subject of Auricular Acupuncture.

(Refer to ear diagram for points)

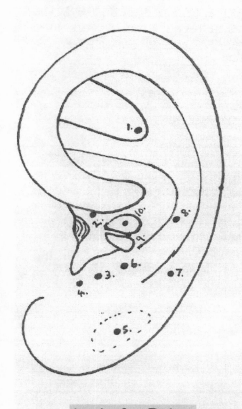

Auricular Points

(1)	Shen-men	(6)	Temple
(2)	Mouth	(7)	Mandible
(3)	Forehead	(8)	Neck
(4)	Eye	(9)	Heart
(5)	Cheek	(10)	Lungs

Step: 4

You have heard me say don't miss any steps out when you carry out a Facial treatment, well this is an exception. Not all patients will require work to be carried out on their neck so Step: 4 is used only when it is needed. These are all points that will benefit the patient's neck, helping to reduce puffiness and reduce lines and wrinkle across the neck. GB21 is particularly effective at stimulating the neck muscles and help to strengthen the neck generally. Not all patients require work on the neck area so I will only use these points when there is a particular requirement. (See Diagram: 1)

ST13 Qi Hu (Qi Door) A point used for treating the lungs, if the lungs are working freely tension to the neck muscles will be reduced.

GB21 Jian Jing (Shoulder Well) The point is located on the high point of the Trapezius muscle, and is a powerful valve for unblocking energy, when the smooth flow of energy is achieved in this area the neck becomes less tense and Qi flows freely.

ST9 Ren Ying (People Welcome) In 5 Element practice this point is recognised as a window to the sky point which has a very powerful effect on the patient's mind and spirit. In the context of this treatment we are using the point purely for its attribute regarding the benefits to the throat.

(All points needled bi-laterally)

Step: 5
Working on the head and face

When starting to work on the face and the head I will sit behind the patient and the first point I would needle would be **DU20** Bai Hui (One Hundred meetings). Somewhere in my past I heard this point referred to by the name of Upright Pillar and I will always remember the description that was given by a former tutor as to the use of this point.

It was described to me as the point where you could attach a piece of string and be able to hold the patient upright When things are getting to much for a patient and the pressures of the world are holding them down, this point is a fantastic point to keep them upright. This description has stuck with me and I always like to use this point when I can, in the context of this treatment I am using the point to lift as the whole idea behind this treatment is to lift.

Following on from **DU20** I then needle **BL6** Cheng Guang (Light Guard) needle posterior at an angle and as you do so apply an upward pressure on the patients forehead with your free hand as if you are gently pulling the skin towards the rear of the head, for these points I always use the 1 inch 14 gauge needles. When these needles are securely in place it is time to work on the patient's eyebrow area. Starting with the left brow spread the fingers of your free hand over the brow and gently lift toward the top of the head sliding you fingers up towards the hairline as you do so. Using a 1 inch needle, insert into the point **GB14** which is used in cases where there is Facial paralysis.

We now need to work on the actual eyebrow itself. My needle of preference for this area would be the intradermal needle probably the 6mm size although some practitioners prefer to use a ½" needle. With the intradermal needle I feel I have more accuracy and control, although its use does take a little practice.

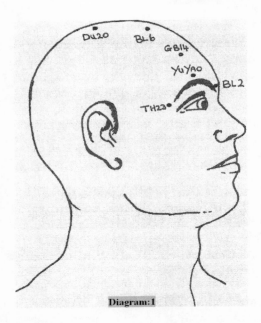

Diagram:1

Lift the medial end of eyebrow and secure the intradermal needle into point **BL2** Zan Shu (Collect bamboo), do the same with the middle of the eyebrow and secure into extra point **YuYao** for those of you not familiar with this point it is an extra point located directly in the middle of the brow, also needle the lateral end of the eye brow into point **SJ23** Zhu Kong (Silk Bamboo Hollow), repeat this procedure firstly left and then right.

When using the intradermal needles always insert with an upward motion, this then ties in with the face lift concept that we are trying to achieve. If you have performed this step of the procedure correctly your patient should have the look of someone raising their eyebrows and who is looking just a little startled. (See Diagram: 1 and photo below)

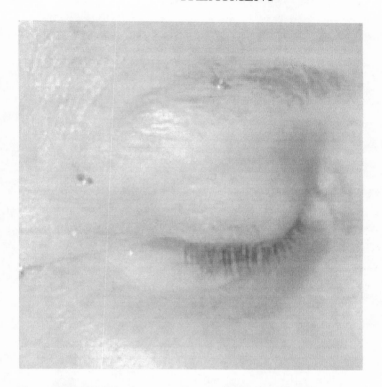

(Intradermal needles inserted into BL2 and Yu Yao)

Step: 6
Needle the chin and cheek areas
Firstly, locate point **ST5** Da Ying (Great Welcome), slightly above this point and approx 1 cun back needle towards the ear and into the cheek. If needled correctly this should produce a grabbing sensation in the cheek muscle, when needling this point the needle will have to be at an approx 45 degree angle to the face.

After needling both left and right sides, move on to the side of the face just below the ear, thread the needle from point **SI17** Tian Rong (Heavenly Appearance) to **SJ17** Yi Feng (Wind Screen) needle with extreme caution, again the grabbing sensation should be achieved. (See Diagram: 2)

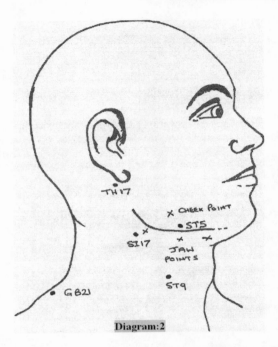

Diagram:2

When I have finished needling these points I usually needle both **Ren 23** Lian Quan (Angle Spring) and **Ren 24** Cheng Jiang (Receiving Fluid) again using an evens technique.

The practitioner now needs to look at their patient's face and pick three symmetrical points on either side of the jaw. The first of these points should be directly below **ST5** Da Ying (Great Welcome). The needles that we are using now are not inserted into specific Acupuncture points but are inserted directly below the jaw bone into the muscle. As this technique is carried out apply some downward pressure as if you were tucking and pinning the skin under the jaw bone. (See Diagram: 2 for point locations). This description sounds very dramatic but what we are trying to achieve is a stimulation of the muscle in the upper neck to help get rid of the jowls that most of us complain about.

For all of the points described in this step I am using the 1 inch 14 gauge needles. It must be stressed that my needle technique is light compared to many other traditions of

36

THE FACIAL ENHANCEMENT ACUPUNCTURE 10 STEPS
TREATMENT

Acupuncture needling and this should, in my opinion, always be the case when working with the face I would much rather take a little longer over treatments and try to ensure as little discomfort to the patient as possible.

Step: 7
At this stage I like to check the control needles in the patient's hand and arm and give them a slight stimulation to aid with any pain relief.

From my experience I have not had any patients who have complained of any discomfort during a treatment. Checking the needles at this stage allows me to get up and stretch my legs and take the patients pulses, if I feel it useful to do so.

Step: 8
Front of Face
For the points that I am about to describe I would generally use the half inch needles. Firstly needle **ST4** Di Cang (Earth Granary) a very important point that can be used to aid conditions of facial paralysis. This point works directly with the muscles of the face. Needle both left and right in the direction of an upward smile this action stimulates the muscles responsible for the smile the Zygomaticus major and Zygomaticus minor muscles and lifts the corner of the mouth.

Needle **LI19** He Liao (Grain Bone) using evens technique near to the side of the nose at the top end of the Nasal labial groove, which is the indent that runs from the side of the mouth up until the side of the nose.

ST3 Ju Liao (Great Cheekbone) and **SI18** Quan Liao (Cheek Bone) are next to each other on the lower part of the cheek. As their name suggests these points are used for the benefits they give to the cheek area of the patient. Needle in an upwards direction into these points they form the basis of sculpting the cheek shape. The results that I have achieved with these points are probably some of the most dramatic and they are amongst my favorite Acupuncture points on the face.

You will be amazed at the definition that can be achieved on a patient's face by the regular stimulation of these points. (See Diagram: 3)

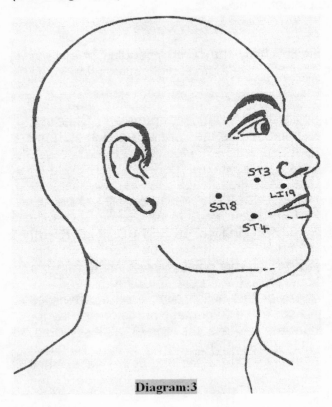

Diagram:3

Step: 9
Intradermal needling

Up until this point the needle techniques and the Acupuncture points we have been using have all been very familiar to us.

We are now going to look at using intradermal needles. Until I started experimenting with Facial techniques they were a new product to me, now I would not be without them. They are the most versatile of needles and I have used them in everyday practice for conditions such as frozen shoulder and lower back pain. The needles that I like to use are a

THE FACIAL ENHANCEMENT ACUPUNCTURE 10 STEPS
TREATMENT

Japanese brand that are either 3mm or 6mm in length and come individually packaged.

The only way to really successfully insert these needles is to use a good pair of surgical tweezers it is also useful to have that magnet handy just in case you drop a needle during a treatment.

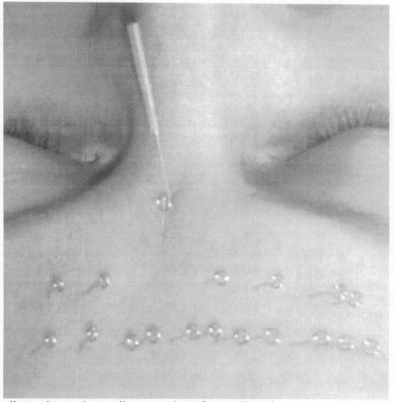

(Intradermal needles used on frown lines)

The principle behind the technique I use with the intradermals is very similar to that which some practitioners know as threading needles. The intradermals are inserted at a slight angle, approx 60 degrees along lines on the face that we want to encourage to fade and fill out naturally. These can be the frown lines on the forehead and the grooves between the eyebrows (The number elevens as one patient calls them). I also use these needles in the nasal labial groove that we talked about earlier as well as the fine lines and wrinkles around the eye (See Diagram: 4). Another common area for treatment with these needles are the lines that appear around patients lips especially people who have been quite heavy smokers.

The intradermal needles should be inserted along the lines at gaps of no more than a couple of millimeters, as you can imagine depending on the patient you will get through quite a few packets of these needles. When you start to use this technique of needling it will feel very strange to you, as like me you have more than likely been taught to use as little intervention as possible when practicing Acupuncture.

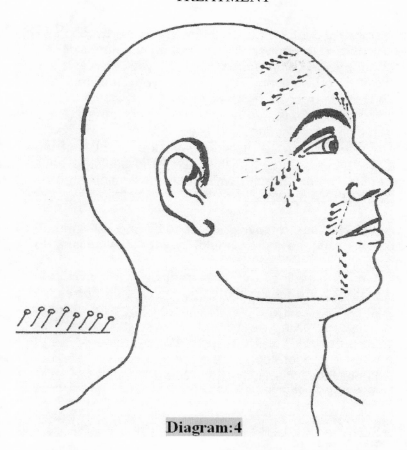

Diagram:4

Be patient and take your time when using these needles and you will find the results are well worth the effort. I find this part of the treatment the most enjoyable as it allows the practitioner to be artistic and flexible in their approach. The practitioner can explore each patient's face and treat individual characteristics that are particular to that patient alone. The results that can be achieved using these needles are fantastic and I would urge practitioners to experiment with them further in other areas of their practice. At this stage of the treatment I like to leave my patients to relax for approx 15 minutes. I usually write my notes up and let them listen to some relaxing music. When I am ready to continue again I will start to remove the needles.

Firstly remove the intradermal needles using the tweezers; a useful tip here is to apply pressure to the skin alongside the intradermal needle using a cotton bud as you remove it this helps prevent bruising and also means you can stem any drops of blood as soon as they form. When all of the intradermal needles have been removed I work from the top down removing the Acupuncture needles in reverse order to which they were inserted, finishing with the needles of the feet. If any bruises appear at this stage it is useful to have some arnica cream on hand which can be administered as soon as the bruise appears.

If you take your time removing the needles and use the cotton bud as described there should be very little bruising to contend with.

When all of the needles have been removed check with the patient that they are feeling okay and check their pulses. At this stage we have finished the treatment. However, I like to finalise things by giving my patient a Facial massage. This usually lasts about 10 to 15 minutes and is an ideal time to relax and have a good look and, more importantly, a feel of your patients face; this is the time when I plan what I will work on for their next visit.

Step: 10
The Facial massage
I cannot profess to being a qualified masseur. The techniques that I employ have come about through experimentation and by having Facial massages myself of which I am a great fan. The main aim of this step is to finalise the treatment that we have performed and to send the patient away feeling renewed and relaxed. It is also an ideal opportunity to look at the work that you have carried out and plan what you would like to do for the next treatment.

The Facial massage can be as long or as short as you feel you want to do. Perhaps it is something that you do not want to get involved with at all; it is entirely up to you. However, I do recommend that you finish with a Facial massage of some sort. When I started doing these treatments I read a lot about aromatherapy techniques and oils and purchased some ready blended oils which are ideal for what we are trying to do. As I progressed I started to blend my own oils and creams and also started to research into the subject of Indian head and face massage.

I have found that my patients really enjoy this part of the treatment and it has really been worth my time and effort to investigate ways of improving this treatment for them. If you spend sometime investigating what works for you then I believe it will be time well spent. When you start to look into Facial massage as a subject in its own right you find that there are many books written on the subject and many practitioners who specialize in this type of treatment. Working with the Facial muscles of a patient using massage has, for a long time, been recognised as a way of delaying the ageing process and improving the patient's Facial appearance.

If you then consider that with Acupuncture we are working with those same muscle groups but to a far greater depth than just massage then it is hardly surprising that we should be getting such good results. I will go through a few of the massage techniques that I use and then leave it up to you to do your own investigation what I am about to describe here should be enough to get you going. Once the patient is relaxed, start by using gentle acupressure to the point DU20 and the same pressure to points BL6 and GB14 this gentle pressure stimulates the point and helps to relax the patient.

Using a massage oil or cream gently smooth out the area of the patient's neckline and jaw, always working with an upward motion and always with very gentle yet deliberate pressure. When massaging the face, I find it's good to follow the areas that I have previously needled i.e. along the nasal labial line and the area around the eyes and always pay special care to this are as the eyes are very sensitive.

Apply light pressure with the pad of your finger to the points ST2 and ST3 and also SI18. When you have finished this area pay special attention to the jaw line and using an upward stroking technique gently massage the area of the lower cheek down to the mandible bone of the jaw.

The thing to remember about any massage technique is that you cannot do any harm at all, it is just about the level of good that you can do. Your patient will respond to even the slightest massage technique but as you improve and your technique develops you will find this part of the treatment both rewarding to you and to your patient.

3
The End (Or Perhaps the Beginning)

Well that's it, that's a full Facial Enhancement Acupuncture treatment. What happens now is that generally the patient leaps up and makes a beeline straight to the mirror, although not ideal, you will have the devil of a job to stop them. What you must point out to them is at this stage there has been an awful lot going on and it will probably be better to look at their face when the skin has had time to settle down.

I hope you have enjoyed this introduction to a type of Acupuncture that is rapidly growing in the West. Facial Enhancement Acupuncture may not be everyone's idea of why they trained to be an acupuncturist, but my view is that patients are going to always want this type of procedure and I would much rather someone who has trained long and hard as we Acupuncturists do, be responsible for carrying it out. For those of us in the profession, we know how wondrous and powerful Acupuncture can be so why not let our patients experience it from every perspective. What I would like to emphasise is that if your patient is not balanced on the inside then whatever you do to their appearance they will never be happy. Now that's where we come in as Traditional Acupuncturists. We can do something about the inner balance as well, that is the advantage we have over so many so called beauty therapies.

THE POCKET GUIDE TO FACIAL ENHANCEMENT ACUPUNCTURE

If you have decided that perhaps this type of Acupuncture is not for you then that's fine. I would like to thank you for your interest and hope you have enjoyed what you have read.

If however you are like me and excited about offering a fantastic new treatment to your patients then good luck, and go for it, remember people will always be looking for something to make them look and feel better so why not let something as wonderful as Acupuncture help them.

Document Templates

The Following documents are examples of some of the leaflets that I use in my practice, the practitioner disclaimer form is particularly useful and you are welcome to adapt and utilise it for use in your own clinic.

- Patient disclaimer form
- Sample patients guide leaflet
- Sample patient incentive offer

Sample Disclaimer form

The Mitchell Hill Clinic

Facial Enhancement Acupuncture

Paul Adkins.Lic.Ac.BA(Hons)FEA.MBAcC

Facial Enhancement Acupuncture Treatment – Patient Disclaimer.

I hereby understand that by its very nature, Acupuncture and other forms of Chinese Medicine, (including but not exclusive to, Acupuncture, acupressure, massage, herbs, aromatherapy, direct and indirect moxibustion, cupping, and electrical stimulation), may cause minor discomfort and may irritate the skin or leave a mark, bruise, or burn. I have been made aware of the risks involved and agree to receive treatment as discussed totally at my own risk. I acknowledge that no claims, promises, or guarantees are being made as to the risk and effectiveness of any treatment and therefore accept full responsibility for the outcome of said treatment.

Patient's name:................................

Signature:.............................   Date:........................

46

THE END (OR PERHAPS THE BEGINNING)

Advertising Leaflet
A Patients' Guide
Facial Enhancement Acupuncture
What is it?
Facial Enhancement is not the latest fad or new thing on the market. It has, in fact, been practiced in China for thousands of years. It is Acupuncture on points of the face to stimulate the meridians and therefore improve muscle tone and skin contraction, this in turn helps to eliminate fine lines and wrinkles. The treatment also reduces the sagging jowls and helps to eliminate puffiness by improving the metabolism - the skin circulation is greatly improved and this helps even out color tone and tightens the pores. As the treatment is totally natural and is working with the body's energy, the patient will feel revitalized all over and their general sense of well being will be improved - this is a fantastic alternative to medical and chemical treatments.

What is involved?
Improvements can be evident after the first treatment, although significant improvements are usually clearer after the patient has received a number of treatments.
It is completely up to you the patient you may decide you would like a few treatments during the build up to a special occasion or you may want to embark on regular treatments throughout the year, it's up to you.

Does it hurt?
The needles that are used for Acupuncture are very fine disposable needles. There is very little sensation when needled with them and only a mild stinging sensation may be experienced on some occasions, in fact the whole experience of a treatment can be very relaxing in itself.

Who carries out the Treatment?
Paul Adkins is a Traditional Acupuncturist who is qualified in 5 Element Acupuncture and also the developer of Facial Enhancement Acupuncture. He has always had a fascination with the Orient

47

and Chinese medicine and is a 1st Dan martial artist. Paul is the proprietor of the Mitchell Hill Clinic in Truro and is fully registered and insured for the practice of Acupuncture. Appointments are available at anytime to discuss the procedure with you further and to assist with any questions that you may have.

To answer any questions or to arrange a Free Consultation please contact:
Paul Adkins.Lic.Ac.BA(Hons)FEA.MBAcC
12 Mitchell Hill
Truro
Cornwall
TR1 1EE

Sample special offer leaflet
Introduce a friend and save on your next treatment
The Mitchell Hill Clinic has been open for business for a few months now and I am overwhelmed with the support and response I have received.I have been introduced to some lovely patients, of which you are one of them, and want to give something back for all your support. I am eager to grow my business from strength to strength, and you may be able to help me with this. If you know of anyone who may have considered Acupuncture, be it traditional or Facial Enhancement, but may be hesitant of the treatment and its results, why not introduce them to me. For every new patient I receive through recommendation, I am offering the recommender the chance to receive their next treatment with a discount of £20 off. I am enclosing a few of my business cards in the hope you may want to spread the word. I am still offering a FREE consultation to anyone who wishes to find out more about how I can help and treat them and what is involved. Once any new patient has received their first treatment, I will offer you your next treatment at the discounted rate, whether it is against your present course of treatment or maybe you would like to try something new.
Once again, thank you for your support.

THE END (OR PERHAPS THE BEGINNING)

I buy all of my needles from these two companies and would highly recommend either of them for your supplies.

Acupuncture Needle suppliers, highly Recommended for Facial supplies

www.harmonymedical.co.uk

Very helpful needle supplier

http://www.balancehealthcare.co.uk

4
References and Bibliography

I have listed many of the publications and journals that I have found of interest during my Acupuncture career to date, I am sure many are well known to you but you may find others that are new and of interest.

Advanced Study in the Health Sciences. (1975) *Acupuncture Anesthesia, A translation of a Chinese Publication of the same title*
1975 p312, 65.144-45.
Washington: U.S.Government printing office.

Birch,S, J. and Felt, R, L. (1999) *Understanding Acupuncture*
1999 p53
New York: Churchill Livingstone.

Chen,K. and Yongqiang,C. (1991) *Handbook to Chinese Auricular therapy*
1991 p99, 107
Beijing: Foreign languages Press.

Chen,J,Y,P. (1973) *Acupuncture Anesthesia in the peoples republic of China,*
United States: Department of Health.

REFERENCES AND BIBLIOGRAPHY

Chi-Lin,Y. (2003) *Acupuncture Anesthesia for a patient with complex Congenital Anomalies*
Volume 13/No2
www.medicalAcupuncture.org

College of Traditional Acupuncture. (2000) *Acupuncture Point Compendium*
Leamington Spa Warwickshire: College of Traditional Acupuncture.

Deadman,P. and Al-Khafaji,M. (2001) *A manual of Acupuncture*
2001 p 99,104,390,399.
England: Journal of Chinese Medicine publications.

Duke,M. (1972) *Acupuncture*
1972 p 105,5,4,2
New York: Pyramid House books.

Eckman,P. (1996) *In the footsteps of the yellow emperor*
1996 p64-65
San Francisco: Cypress book company.

Galston,A,W. *Article and Picture, Abdominal Surgery*
Dispatch News Service

Jianping,L.Yanliang,C. and Rinhua,S. (1990) *Chinese Acupuncture and Moxibustion*
1990 p 74
Shanghai: Publishing house of Shanghai University of Traditional Chinese Medicine.

Kaptchuck,T,J. (1983) *The Web that has no Weaver-understanding Chinese Medicine*
1983 p81
New York: Congdon and Weed

Lewith,G,T. (2003) *Acupuncture its place in Western medical science*
http://www.complemed.co.uk

Lowe, W,C. (1973) *Introduction to Acupuncture Anesthesia*
1973 p73
New York: Medical examination publishing co Inc.

Mere-China. (2003) *Acupressure can serve as pain control in minor traumas*
15th July 2003
www.merechina.com

Mock,YP.(1991) *Medical Acupuncture applications in Surgical Anesthesia.*
www.medicalAcupuncture.org   Spring/1991
The Journal of the American Academy of Medical Acupuncture.

Mock,YP. (2000) *Acupuncture assisted Anesthesia*
www.medicalAcupuncture.org   Spring/Summer 2000 Vol, 12 no 1
The Journal of the American Academy of Medical Acupuncture.

Philippine Council for Agriculture. (2002) *Acupuncture Analgesia in Water Buffalo*
www.agnet.org

Porkert,M. and Ullman,C. (1982) *Chinese Medicine its history, Philosophy and practice*
1st American edition, p229
New York: William Morrow and Co.

Posner,G. (1999) *Chinese Acupuncture for Heart Surgery Anesthesia*
The Scientific review of Alternative Medicine.
www.hcrc.org

Quan,S,X. (1985) *Applied Chinese Acupuncture for Cinical practitioners*
1985 p10
China: Shandong Science and technology Press.

REFERENCES AND BIBLIOGRAPHY

Redmond,Martin,Florence,Barry and Glass. (2003) *Effective analgesic modalities for ambulatory patients*
2003, Vol 21,No 2, p329-46
Anaesthesiology Clinic North America

Renhui, Xin'an, Li,Wanjun,Huifang and Fang. *Acupuncture Anesthesia and combined Acupuncture Anesthesia in war surgery*
Department of Anesthesia, General Hospital of Guangzhou Unit of PLA, Guangzhou

Reston,J. (1971) *Now let me tell you about my appendectomy in Peking*
New York Times Newsbook.

Rosenfeld,I.(1998) *Acupuncture goes mainstream (Almost)*
August 16:1998 p10-11
Parade Magazine.

Schoen,A,M. (1994) *Veterinary Acupuncture Ancient Art to Modern Medicine*
1994 p277-283
USA : Mosby

Schwartz,L. (1998) *Acupuncture Augmentation of local Anesthesia with intravenous sedation for a child undergoing awake Craniotomy*
Spring/Summer 1998 Vol, 10 No 1

www.medicalAcupuncture.org
Cheng,R. (1980) Mechanisms *of electro Acupuncture analgesia as related to endorphins and monoamines; an intricate system is proposed*
Thesis: University of Toronto

Streitberger,K,Dr. (2003) *Acupuncture in Anesthesia*
www.icmart.org

Terra,R,P. (2003) *Anesthesia risks and complication*
January 2003
www.meritcare.com

Veith,I. (1972) *The Yellow Emperors Classic of internal Medicine*
New edition, p 3
Berkeley: University of California press.

Wallnoffer,H. and Rottauscher,A,V. *Chinese folk Medicine and Acupuncture*
P 126-127
New York: Bell publishing company inc.

Wen,Dr. *Acupuncture Anesthesia Protocols*
Orthopaedic surgery on the elbow
China : Yunnan Province Hospital

A Barefoot Doctors Manual. (1985) *Practical Chinese Medicine and Health*
1985 Edition
New York : Gramercy Publishing Company

Academy of Traditional Chinese Medicine. (1975) *an outline of Chinese Acupuncture*
Peking : Foreign Language Press

Chong-hao,Z. (2001) *Effect Of Local Injection Of Steroid And Anaesthetics On Electro Acupuncture:Prevention Of Immediate Analgesia And Induction Of Hyperalgesia*
http://www.medicalAcupuncture.org

Christensen,E. (1998*) Theories on the Effects of Acupuncture on the Nervous System*
http://serendip.brynmawr.edu

Connelly,D,M. (1975) *Traditional Acupuncture The law of the Five Elements*
Maryland : The Centre for Traditional Acupuncture inc

REFERENCES AND BIBLIOGRAPHY

Darwin,C,R. (1997) *The Acupuncture Anesthesia - a biocibernetic technique*
http://www.icmart.org

Devitt,M. (2004) *Treatment Before Surgery Reduces Anxiety in Both Mother and Child*
http://www.Acupuncturetoday.com

Dharmananda,S. (1988) *Pearls from the Golden Cabinet*
USA : Oriental Healing Arts Institute

Feit,R,& Zmiewski,P. (1990) *Acumoxa therapy, Treatment of Disease*
Vol 11
Massachusetts: Paradigm Publications

Gascoigne,S. (2001) *The Clinical Medicine Guide, A Holistic Perspective*
2001 Edition
Ireland : Jigme Press

Gordon,K. (2000) *Acupuncture Analgesia and the Mind-Brain Problem*
http://dubinserver.colorado.edu

Klide,A,M. (1992) *Veterinary Acupuncture Analgesia*
http://www.Acupuncture.com
Koo,ST. (2002) *Acupuncture analgesia in a new rat model of ankle sprain pain.*
http://www.ncbi.nlm.nih.gov

Larre,C. and Rochat de la Vallee,E. (1976) *Survey of Traditional Chinese Medicine*
Maryland : Traditional Acupuncture Institute

Mann,F. (1971) *Acupuncture The Ancient Chinese art of healing and how it works Scientifically*
Revised Edition
New York : Random House

Maciocia,G. (1989) *The Foundations Of Chinese Medicine*
New York : Churchill Livingstone

Maciocia,G. (2000) *Tongue Diagnosis in Chinese Medicine*
5th Edition
Seattle : Eastland Press

Nabeshima,K. (2001) *The Needle and the Sword, health Strategies of a Samurai Acupuncturist*
USA : Kenshi Nabeshima

NCEPOD. (2004) *National confidential enquiry into patient outcome and death*
www.ncepod.org

Rogers,P. (1995) *Acupuncture analgesia for surgery in animals*
http://users.med.

Sekida,K. (1977) *Zen Training, Methods and Philosophy*
1977 4th Edition
Tokyo: Weatherhill

Shanghai University, (1990) *Chinese Acupuncture and Moxibustion*
Shanghai : University of Traditional Chinese Medicine Publishing House

Smith,L,A. *Acupuncture for dental pain*
http://www.jr2.ox.ac.uk

Stener-Victorin,E. (2003) *Electro-Acupuncture as a preoperative analgesic method and its effects on implantation rate and neuropeptide Y concentrations in follicular fluid.*
http://www.ncbi.nlm.nih.gov

Stone,A.(1998) *Acupuncture Anesthesia*
http://beyondwellbeing.com

REFERENCES AND BIBLIOGRAPHY

Stux,G. andPomeranz,B. (1995) *Basics of Acupuncture*
1995 3rd Edition
New York : Springer

Sung,K. (2004) *Acupuncture Analgesia Comparison - Study of Traditional and Sham Acupoint Stimulation*
http://www.ampainsoc.org

Toguchi,M. and Warren,F,Z. (1985) *Complete guide to Acupuncture and Acupressure*
New York : Gramercy Publishing Company

Worsley,J,R. (1998) *Classical Five-Element Acupuncture, The*
Five Elements and the Officials
Vol.111
J.R.&J.B. Worsley

Zhu,M. (1992) *Zhu's Scalp Acupuncture*
Hong Kong : Dragons Publishing

Thank you very much for taking the time to read this guide if you have any questions that I can be of assistance with please contact me via e-mail and I will endeavor to get back to you as soon as I can.
You can contact me at **pointlocation@aol.com**
Best Wishes
Paul

Glossary of Terms

Acuanalgesia: A term that is used in some publications to describe Acupuncture pain relief.

Acupuncture: The insertion of the tips of needles into the skin at specific points for the purpose of treating various disorders by stimulating nerve impulses.

Anaesthetic: A Substance that causes Anesthesia.

Anesthesia: Loss of bodily sensation, and specifically loss of sensation of pain.

Analgesia: An inability to feel pain.

Aspiration: The sucking of fluid or foreign matter into the air passages of the body.

Auricular: Relating to, or received by the sense organs of hearing.

Da-Qi: The sensation that is felt when stimulating an Acupuncture point.

Evens Technique: Needle technique where the needle is inserted vertical and no stimulation is applied to the needle.

Intradermal: Small needle that is used for fine work.

Meridian: Channels through which vital energy is believed to circulate around the body.

N.H.S.: National Health Service.

Postoperative: Occurring in the period following a surgical procedure.

Preoperative: The period before a surgical procedure is undertaken.

Qi: Vital energy believed to circulate around the body in currents.

There are a few pages left blank at the back of the book, I am not one for normally condoning writing in books but you may find it useful to make some notes as you do your first few treatments.

Notes

GLOSSARY OF TERMS

<u>Notes</u>

Made in the USA